Dimensions
of
Humanistic
Medicine

ESSAYS IN HUMANISTIC MEDICINE

Dimensions of Humanistic Medicine

Reflections on Science and Technology,
Patient Care, Administration,
Training and Health Policy

Stuart Miller, Ph. D.
Naomi Remen, M.D.
Allen Barbour, M.D.
Marguerite Abell Nakles, R.N.
Sara Miller, M.A.
Dale Garell, M.D.

THE INSTITUTE FOR
THE STUDY OF HUMANISTIC MEDICINE

© 1975. The Institute for the Study of Humanistic Medicine. All rights reserved. The Institute conducts the Program in Humanistic Medicine in affiliation with Mt. Zion Hospital and Medical Center, San Francisco, California. The work of the Institute is supported by Contract No. 1-MB-44200, Bureau of Health Resources Development, Department of Health, Education and Welfare, and by grants from the Mary Reynolds Babcock Foundation, the Benjamin Rosenthal Foundation, the Andrew Norman Fund, Mr. Donald Flaxman, Mrs. Patience Hite, Mrs. Katherine Tremaine, Film Corporation of America and Mr. Martin J. Farber.

❖❖

Additional copies of volumes in the series, "Essays in Humanistic Medicine" are available from the Institute for the Study of Humanistic Medicine, 3847 Twenty-First Street, San Francisco, California 94114. Costs are $4.00 each, to cover expenses of printing, handling and postage, for *Case Studies and Methods in Humanistic Medical Care* and the *Masculine Principle, the Feminine Principle and Humanistic Medicine;* $5.00 for *Dimensions of Humanistic Medicine.*

CONTENTS

PREFACE

Concern for the human quality of health care is an increasingly wide-spread preoccupation. Health professionals and the general public alike express with increasing vigor their desire to see the health care system evolve along more fully humanistic lines. This short volume is intended to suggest some of the principal areas for thinking and action toward such a new medicine: patient care, the humanization of science and technology, administration, professional training and health policy. Clearly, these five are not all the necessary dimensions of a humanistic medical evolution. Nor are these preliminary thoughts meant to be exhaustive or definitive. Systematic work on a national scale toward the large goal is just beginning. It must be stressed, however, that if a comprehensive humanistic medicine is to evolve, the medical system must be examined in a comprehensive fashion. No narrow concentration on any one important element in the health care system — be it nursing, or the education of physicians, or health policy — will be enough.

The six papers published here also provide a brief introduction to the work of the Institute for the Study of Humanistic Medicine during its first three years. Interested readers can further pursue some of these ideas in publications of the Institute already printed or in preparation.

A word about the genesis of these papers will be useful in explaining their tone and form. They were originally written to be spoken, as contributions to the Conference "Alternative Futures for Medicine," held at Airlie house in the Spring of 1975. This meeting of health policy planners, congressional staff experts on health, directors of federal offices and programs, research scientists, physicians, administrators, nurses, and educators was itself important testimony to the widely perceived need for a new look at the health care system. The staff members who authored the papers were invited by Rick J. Carlson, the Conference director, to present the work-to-date of this Institute as it might bear on some of the larger issues of health policy.

Although we did not explicitly state this position, we do believe that the major problems facing medicine are either fundamentally or in large part problems of an inadequately humanistic conceptualization and practical implementation of the elements of the health care system. If one looks at malpractice, the yet unconquered "diseases of civilization" like heart disease, cancer and high blood pressure, or the shortage of health care resources — to take a few major examples, it seems clear that none of these major problems can be solved without serious attention to the concerns of humanism in medicine. Malpractice claims arise in part because physicians are not fully trusted by their patients; the diseases of civilization arise in some measure from our inability to help patients adequately understand and then change lifestyles which endanger health; and the shortage of health resources arises, in part, from our inattention to ways of using "consumers" as responsible and active "providers" of health care. This short volume was never directed to such heights of theoretical analysis. However, the interested reader may look for his own support of this position in his experience within the medical system and sometimes within the chapters below.

These chapters on dimensions of humanistic medicine were edited by myself and Dr. Naomi Remen. This volume is dedicated to Rick Carlson and the vast numbers of health professionals and others who daily work to realize in practice the vision of a more fully humanistic medicine.

Stuart Miller
Director
Institute for the Study of Humanistic Medicine

Chapter I

Introduction:
The Present Cultural Crisis and the Need for a Humanistic Medicine

Stuart Miller, Ph.D.

This paper concerns an important dimension of humanistic medicine: awareness of the larger cultural context which is essential to a true perspective on the problems of health care. Reviewing this context points to the need for and the practicability of systematic medical innovation toward humanistic goals.

It is commonplace of contemporary social criticism to say that the major cultural problem of our century, and perhaps of the next one too, is the integration of our new materialistic science with the full range of man's human needs — needs for common caring, all the way to needs for cosmic understanding. The well-known problems of dehumanization in health care are, of course, part of this larger problem. Man's scientific and technological capacity has apparently out-raced his ability to integrate it with other aspects of his humanness. Whether we look to politics and the bomb, or the environment and pollution, or education and its harsh sterilities — to whatever field we turn — the problem is the same: How do we reconcile our magnificent scientific and material capabilities with our other human concerns and needs?

At the very highest levels of scientific achievement, however, the problem of science versus man dissolves. An Einstein has no problem reconciling science and wonder, science and religion, science and compassion, science and a deep sense of the interpenetrating wholeness of all things. As Dr. LeShan has pointed out, the great physicists and the great mystics frequently saw the same unified vision and differ only in the descriptive language they have used. The mystical oriental text, the Dammapadha, says that the material world is not entirely separate from the human mind. So, for example, does the physicist Percy Bridgman. "In general," says Bridgman, "we should never think of the world around us without also thinking of the nervous machinery in our heads, by means of which we acquire knowledge of the world."[1] Such parallel quotations of physicists and religious leaders could be multiplied to show there is no necessary conflict between materialistic science and man's so-called "softer" aspects. At the pinnacles of intellect and insight, man and the material world of science are apparently united.

Though this truth is comforting for those of us in the plains and valleys of human life, it is not sufficient for daily living in today's world. I suspect that even great scientists, with their scientomystical glimpses of the biggest truth, have their problems with the everyday dehumanization of our institutions, including the institution of medicine. The puzzling thing is that relatively little of a systematic nature — should one say of a scientific nature — is being done to deal with these well-known problems of dehumanization. And yet, as we have seen, it is broadly admitted that the synthesis of science with human needs in every field is the essential problem for human civilization.

Why so little systematic work is being done to resolve these problems is too complex a question to fully answer here, but I would suggest two of the main reasons are these: First, it is commonly believed that nothing conscious can be done about dehumanization — that is, it is felt that we cannot increase our humanness by deliberate efforts. Either we've got it or we haven't. To take medicine as an example, either a doctor is a caring person, or he isn't; either a doctor has a "feel" for the human values of his patients, or he hasn't.

A second reason that problems of dehumanization are not systematically approached, is that professionals within a given field tend to believe that other professionals are not really interested in such things. In medicine, for example, so apparently exclusive is the professional interest in "hard fact," in competency, in efficient production and responsible management, that the average medical professional believes that no one else is interested in such complementary concerns as will be discussed in the following papers: the meaning of illness, the experience of pain and suffering, or the professional's ability to help a patient realize inner dignity and strength. Consequently, the health professional is often loathe to discuss these matters with colleagues and this leads to a lack of open communication and concerted action.

The work of the Institute for the Study of Humanistic Medicine was started some three years ago, with the belief that something deliberate *could* be done about dehumanization in the health care field. This belief was founded on the Directors' previous work in education. With support from the Ford Foundation and the University of California at Santa Barbara, a group of educators, working over several years, had shown that practical methods for humanizing public school education could, indeed, be developed and integrated within the existing educational system.[2] We believed that cognate methods could be found to counter the parallel problems of dehumanization in the health care field.

Accordingly, we recruited a group of fifteen medical professionals who agreed to commit themselves to a personal and professional exploration of what we called — for want of a better term — humanistic medicine. We hoped to explore a medicine that was not just responsive to the body of the patient, but also to his *feelings*, his *mind*, his *will*, his *imagination*, his *creativity*, his *aspirations*, his *values*, his capacity for making *ethical choices* — in short, a medicine responsive to the whole human life of the person who is a patient. We proposed a demanding exploration of many years' duration, involving several evenings per month, a dozen weekends a year, and daily studying, writing, and thinking.[3] In addition, there was a demand that the health professional group be prepared to invest their own humanity in the search; for if modern medicine is to practically acknowledge human feeling, health professionals are going to have to explore feelings, including their own, in order to find methods of restoring feeling to medicine in appropriate ways. If modern medicine is to recognize the patient's need to engage with the questions of life value evoked by illness, health professionals are going to have to explore life values, including their own, in order to find ways to restore these values to medicine. It would be a demanding process, and we expected that only a few volunteers would be interested.

Instead, we received hundreds of applications — not only from California, but from states as distant as Massachusetts, and from countries as remote as the Netherlands. This large, though latent, interest in humanistic medicine was an important discovery — one buttressed by 150 intensive interviews we conducted with applicants to the Program. A curious aspect of these interviews was the frequent expectation of interviewees that many of their immediate colleagues would not share their interests. In many instances, Dr. Jones would tell us that he himself was concerned with the implementation of humanistic values in medicine, but that Smith would never be interested. And Smith was typical of course. It happened half a dozen times, while listening to such claims, that we would know we would be interviewing Smith on the following night.

Experience since those early days confirms the existence of a latent but widespread longing among health care people for a change in the system. This finding should not be surprising. One cannot believe that people elect to endure the grueling apprenticeship of the health professions without an underlying motive of deep human caring and concern, a desire to probe the mysteries of pain, suffering and death — without a truly scientific desire to know man as he is, that is to say, as a whole. And yet, despite these motives and goals, workers tend to find themselves in increasingly regimented, technologized, specialized and routinized professional lives, often marked by narrow gauge interchanges with both patients and colleagues. Is it any wonder that a deep frustration, much of it unconscious, may be expressed as hunger for a common substitute for human experience and knowledge — money and the matter that it can buy? The public recurrently criticizes certain health professionals for their materialism. But I submit that underneath the increasingly material and materialistic facade of contemporary health care, is a longing for a more humanistic practice that does not yet know how to express itself, for which ways and methods have not yet been made clear.

Frequently, there is a fear that to restore humanness to medicine would be to lose scientific rigor, technical efficiency and objective judgment. We have not found this to be a realistic fear. The fifteen professionals with whom we have, for three years, explored humanistic innovations in health care, have not found humanism and science to be irreconcilable in practice. By reintroducing largely neglected aspects of the person into the health care transaction — aspects like feelings, meaning, the creative use of illness, the spirit — our staff find that the effectiveness of the traditional health care of the body increases. In a complementary way, medicine's particular focus on the body tends to illuminate our knowledge of human meaning, feelings, and values. As Dr. Pellegrino has pointed out, medicine is, by its nature, the most scientific of the humanities.[4]

❖ ❖ ❖

Experience indicates that medicine is a human art that can be increasingly understood and learned. What is needed is the *will* to learn it — the will to reconcile science and human needs, to go through the laborious and lengthy process of finding the methods of reconciliation. Our work in the Institute is only beginning. The task of implementing humanness in a scientific age is not going to be a short one.

Fortunately, as Dr. Garell discusses below, the large work of systematically reconciling scientific medicine with human values is beginning in many quarters and many are engaged in the task. The result of that work will surely be a better, richer, and more realistic medicine. The following papers give an indication of the hard realities of this work in a variety of day-to-day situations. We have found that practical humanistic innovation is difficult work, requiring time, patience, and courage, but we have also found that it is possible to take practical steps toward a realistic transformation of contemporary medicine. We look forward to the emergence of a new medicine that has all the power contemporary science, technology and administrative organization have brought to the medical enterprise — in addition to having the human wholeness which can make that power more sensitive and humanly effective.

Chapter II

Humanistic Patient Care:
Toward a Contemporary Synthesis
of the Art and Science
# of Medicine

Naomi Remen, M.D.

*To be practically relevant, a concern for humanism in
medicine must address itself to new ways of conceiving
and practicing patient care. This paper begins to introduce
a model for a more humanistic conception of the patient
and the physician. The general discussion and the case have
broad application to such current issues as hospitalization
versus ambulatory care and patient rights, among others.*

In the last fifty years, medicine has acquired vast new scientific and technological knowledge. This new learning has enabled the profession to be, in many ways, much more effective in the treatment of diseases. In other ways, we are less effective than our colleagues of fifty years ago: less effective in our treatment of the people who have the diseases. The attempt to develop a humanistic medicine addresses itself to this paradox and seeks to reincorporate the "art of medicine" into contemporary patient care. By the art of medicine, I do not mean manner or individual style. Rather, I mean the underlying philosophy and ethical technique: the context and methodology in which we set and apply the scientific process of medicine.

During the past fifty years, the art of medicine has gradually become separated from the science of medicine. Modern physicians increasingly tend to serve their patients with science alone. But while patients acknowledge the value of scientific care, they are increasingly more discontent, more critical and even more hostile about their medical care than ever before.

There are many indications that it is the separation of the art from the science of medicine which underlies much of the well-known consumer discontent. The science of medicine has helped patients physically, but it has not satisfied some other essential human needs: needs for personal recognition, compassion, choice and self-determination. These are needs we all share. It would seem reasonable, then, to resynthesize the art of medicine into technological patient care, in order to meet such needs.

In the last half century, however, much has been learned about "human-ness"; much more is understood than formerly, about consciousness, about awareness, about adaptation and communication. Accordingly, the art of medicine which needs synthesizing into care ought to be a new art — as sophisticated and effective as the science it will meet and wed. Fortunately, enough is now known about human process — the development of the individual human being — to enable us to consider formal means of developing and teaching a new art of medicine to those in training.

In the past, this human aspect of care was often left to chance by the professional schools. Either a student learned it from watching others or he didn't. Humanism in medicine was frequently philosophized about but not acted upon. Even now, few schools formally incorporate courses in the practical application of humanistic attitudes into their curricula. Few schools take real responsibility for actively teaching this art, or hold students responsible for meeting standards of practice with regard to this dimension of patient care. It must even be admitted, as Dr. Miller has implied, that few schools recognize a formal and deliberate approach to humanistic care is possible. And yet an awareness of this possibility and a willingness to implement it is important to the emergence of a new synthesis in medicine.

A first step in this direction would be the identification and elaboration of some basic principles of humanistic patient care. Such a paradigm or working definition promotes the rethinking of the daily practice of medicine including alterations in the relationships and roles of both doctor and patient. The expanded paradigm of care can also facilitate efforts to develop ways of teaching a contemporary art of medicine which is synthesized with science.

I would like to describe a case that illustrates some of these principles of patient care. This case concerns a health problem which American physicians face every day. But it also has a personal importance for me. It represents the first time that I had the courage to try some new approaches in my own attempt to practice a more humanistic medicine. At the time that I cared for this patient, my general views of medicine had started to change, but I did not yet trust the new approaches I had been studying. I have since used these and other methods many times and have found that this patient's response to these approaches is typical of other adolescent patients.[1]

❖ ❖ ❖

I first met Harold in the spring of 1973 when he was 13½ years old. My relationship with him began through a phone call from his physician requesting that I accept Harold for admission to our university hospital. There seemed to be no other way to manage his problem. Although I had not yet seen Harold myself, he was well known to the hospital, having been admitted twice in the last two years. During both admissions, he presented with progressive obesity and vague muscle pains. Both times he received an extensive evaluation, including a psychiatric evaluation, and all his studies were normal. He had left the hospital without a diagnosis and had continued to gain weight until he was bedridden and totally isolated from people outside his immediate family. His physician had become desperate: on four different occasions he and others had attempted to put Harold on a diet. All of these diets had failed and Harold had continued to gain. His weight was now such that he might soon develop difficulty in breathing. His physician had phoned me to suggest that I accept Harold as a case of "malignant obesity" — and institute therapy. He proposed that Harold be hospitalized for a period of several months, and placed on a stringent diet which could be enforced by hospital personnel. Part of me agreed: this was what I had been taught was reasonable management of such a situation. But something made me hesitate, and I asked if I could meet Harold and his family first. His physician agreed.

About a week later, Harold and his mother came to see me in my office. I examined him and reviewed his lab data. Although all of his tests were normal, both his pCO_2 and his glucose tolerance were at the upper limits of their accepted values. Harold was 5'3" and weighed almost 210 pounds. He seemed barely alive. He did not walk and made no effort to help us as we struggled to get him from the wheelchair to the scale and back.

I felt overwhelmed. Some of the *diseases of the medical profession* had begun to affect me. Like many other doctors, I was very invested in succeeding, very responsible, and very competitive. I began to feel anxious. Would I succeed in making this patient lose weight? Would I prove myself superior to other doctors who had failed in the "management" of this patient? Momentarily I had taken full control and accepted full responsibility for the outcome. If Harold lost weight, I would take all the credit. If he didn't lose weight, I would take all the blame. Somehow, I was more central in the situation than Harold was.

These feelings lasted until I sat down at my desk and began to talk with Harold. Harold's body was passive and inert, but Harold himself wasn't. Harold was very, very angry and his anger seemed directed at me. The strength and force of his anger surprised me. I realized that I didn't need to be responsible for moving Harold. He had all the strength he needed to move himself. I could be responsible for putting him in touch with his own strength and guiding him as he learned to use it positively. I began to feel more at ease.

For several months I had been studying techniques that might help Harold positively experience his strength and allow me to collaborate with this strength. It seemed to me that Harold needed to experience himself as I experienced him. He needed to experience himself as different from his fat, not heavy and inert, but strong and angry.

I had also recently begun to recognize that illness was often a sort of body language, a way of expressing something. Perhaps Harold's fat had a meaning for him, was some sort of a message to himself or to others. *If he could experience himself as different from his fat, maybe he could read and understand the message that might be in his fat.* I had recently been experientially trained in *inner dialogue,* a technique I had found personally useful in stopping smoking. I decided to use this technique with Harold.

I took a deep breath and came from behind my desk. I took a straight chair from the corner and put in in front of Harold.

"See this chair? Put your fat on it."

"What?"

"Put your fat here. Do you see it in a heap?" I piled it up in an imaginary heap with my hands. Fantasy is an important part of the successful use of inner dialogue. I was counting on Harold's being close enough to childhood to be able to fantasize. Harold started to laugh. He couldn't believe an adult was really saying this to him. He said, "Yup, I see it."

"Talk to it," I said. He laughed again. For the first time, he didn't seem angry.

"What do I say?"

"Tell your fat what you don't like about it." This was easy. Resentment after resentment poured out, ranging from, "I don't have any friends," to "I look ugly." When he finished talking to his fat, I said, "Okay, now tell your fat what you like about it."

"I don't know what you mean."

"Well, what do you get to do that you wouldn't get to do without your fat? Tell your fat." This took longer. Finally, Harold responded: "I don't have to do chores. I don't have to go to school. Mom waits on me. I don't have to play sports. If I played sports, maybe I'd lose."

"Harold," I said, "Who has been saying all these things?"

Harold did what many adolescents do when they catch an adult asking a silly question. With elaborate condescension, he said, "Why, I have been talking, of course."

"Oh," I said, "Is the I that has been talking fat or thin?"

That was a long minute. Finally Harold solved it very simply.

"My fat is there on the chair," he said. "The I that has been talking is thin," and he giggled.

I moved my chair so we were sitting next to each other. "What does thin-you think about your fat?"

"I don't like carrying it. I'm tired of carrying it. I want to put it down. I want to make it go away." So we spent the next few minutes talking about choice and decision. I asked Harold if he had ever had the chance to make an adult decision, one that he made because he wanted to and not because someone else wanted him to. He said that people decided for him. I said, "That's often the way it is with children." I suggested that a decision like losing his fat might be his first opportunity to make a decision as an adult. We also discussed what a consultant was. If Harold made an adult decision, he might also choose to consult with someone else who has special knowledge. That consultant would then make information available to Harold that Harold could use to reach his goal. I was such a consultant. Our clinic nutritionist could be such a consultant. This really interested him. I then suggested that adult decisions required careful thought. I asked him to go home and decide whether he wanted to lose his fat now. If he did, I asked him to call for an appointment.

In two weeks he was back. He had chosen. He wanted to lose weight. He had also written down a lot of questions which would give him the information he needed to know from both his consultants.

Harold's long term follow-up was relatively easy. I saw him for 15 or 20 minutes each week. We decided to discontinue pain medications as they had never helped much. Harold attributed his muscle pain to the burden his fat was placing on his body. He no longer focused on his pain and planned to see if it was a problem after he lost weight. I continued to keep him in touch with the ongoing dialogue between his fat and his thin self. I pointed out how cleverly his fat self would outwit his thin self, or how strong his thin self had been during a big dinner. I stressed this cleverness and strength — these were Harold's qualities. He began to enjoy watching his process and he started to keep a written record of his inner dialogue. Through this process, he eventually realized that he had mistakenly felt that "Big was Strong," and that his fat was his way of saying, "I want to be strong." Once he had read this message, he was able to experience his strength in his ability to decide and choose, rather than in his physical size. His fat no longer seemed necessary to him.

We did have relapses, of course. Occasionally Harold would stop losing weight and become angry and surly. Occasionally I would relapse into a success-failure model and become anxious. Mostly I remember our visits with pleasure — as he does.

At present Harold has been free from muscle pain for almost a year. He goes to school and, because of the demands on his time, he has decided to see me only once a year for check-ups.

Harold ultimately lost almost 100 pounds. I am sure that by hospitalizing him and policing him, he would have lost as much weight. In the past, I would have done this because I would not have had any available alternative. However, I think that what Harold gained through the approach I used is as important as the weight he lost. He has a sense of himself, of his strength, and his ability to choose.

❖ ❖

Harold's case illustrates some of the principles that seem important for the development of a more fully humanistic paradigm of care.[2] One basic principle would be the acknowledgement that *the patient is more than his body and therefore more than his disease.* Having this perspective available, enabled me to help Harold recognize that he was strong and able to change, although he appeared massive and inert. Through *my* awareness of the difference between Harold and his body, I was able to help Harold experience *himself* as different from his fat.

A paradigm of humanistic care should also include the recognition of the *potential opportunity of illness.* The concept of illness is socially and culturally defined as a negative experience — at the least, a nuisance; at the most, a disaster. However, a more humanistic definition of illness would suggest that illness may also be used creatively: as an opportunity to experience identity, strength and personal meaning. As a physician acting from this broader definition, I was able to work with Harold as he redefined his illness for himself. What Harold learned through his obesity may be of use to him in living his life. This points to another principle that deserves a place in a new paradigm of care: *Illness can only be thoroughly defined within the context of the life span of an individual.*

Harold's illness achieved a positive meaning for him within this context.

That the professional and patient are colleagues is another important principle that deserves consideration in a future paradigm of medical care. This relationship provides a basis for the physician to help the patient activate latent psychological, spiritual and biological resources. I was able to establish Harold as a colleague and collaborated with him. But without an awareness of the possibility of collaboration and sharing of responsibility, it is very possible that I might have fallen into my older pattern and engaged, instead, in a power struggle with Harold. In my effort to force him to lose weight, I could well have resorted to an authoritarian, expensive, unnecessary and possibly, in the long run, ineffective hospitalization. This might have cheated him of the opportunity to transform his illness from a self-limitation to a self-teacher and to grow from the experience.

Naturally, collaboration is not always possible, nor is it appropriate in all medical situations. There are certain highly acute phases of the disease process which require the professional to take full and immediate control of the situation and carry the patient through. But even in these situations, doctor and patient collaborate. Most doctors are aware that if the comatose and severely injured patient is unable to collaborate on a physiological level he will die despite our best efforts and all our technology. We actually can do nothing without the collaboration of the patient.

However, this physical collaboration is only a phase. At the end of this acute phase, when the patient is able to respond consciously, the relationship needs to be renegotiated and collaboration above the physical level begun, thus allowing the evolution of the meaning and educational value of the experience for the patient. Illness may then become, as it did with Harold, an opportunity to re-evaluate priorities, values and behaviors, learn new skills and clarify the importance of human relationship in our lives. The positive potential of illness deserves a wide recognition in the work toward more humanistic modes of practice.

Another way of looking at the collaboration between professional and patient reveals an interesting implication of this approach for the costs of modern medical care. One could say that Harold delivered to himself the number of hours of professional care that he did not require of the hospital health team. It is almost as if Harold, and each of us have an "inner doctor" who can be mobilized, at times, in our own behalf. Harold was enabled to mobilize this inner doctor and become an active member of the health care team. Such humanistic *activation of the patient* seems, therefore, an important principle in a future paradigm of care.

❖ ❖ ❖

A Medicine of Evolution

A general goal of the technological medicine of the last fifty years has been to restore the patient to the *status quo ante,* to his condition prior to the onset of the disease.

This condition was usually defined predominantly in physical terms. The goals of a humanistic medicine, however, include the creative use of illness: the use of the experience of illness to facilitate the patient's growth, self-awareness, and self-responsibility. Within this framework the practitioner can aim to restore the patient to a condition more whole and more evolved than his condition prior to the onset of his disease.

A contemporary synthesis of the science of medicine with a new and effective art of medicine will not be merely a medicine of homeostasis but of evolution; an evolution which parallels the total evolution of the individual, and of man himself.

Chapter III

Humanistic Patient Care
a Comparison of the
Disease Model and the Growth Model

Allen B. Barbour, M.D.

This paper draws on the author's thirty-year experience in the practice of internal medicine and further elaborates a reconception of patient care along humanistic lines. The analysis of the disease model as contrasted with an educational or growth model has implications for mounting concerns about the effectiveness and the proliferating costs of care.

Physicians are trained to think largely in the disease model. People come to us with unpleasant sensations in their bodies, disagreeable moods, troublesome behaviors, and a host of other problems for which they seek our advice. Regardless of the nature of the problem, we generally attempt to fit the person into a model of disease. If there is a *symptom,* our word for the problem described by the person (whom we now call a *patient*), we generally make the assumption of a disease, whether physical or psychological, and we set out to classify the disease in our nomenclature.

Whatever the patient describes is organized and classified as the *present illness* on the physician's chart. So we record the symptoms, examine the patient, perform laboratory and X-ray studies, and almost always make a diagnosis. No matter what reason the patient has for consulting us, we have a medical name for it. Sometimes the condition appears to be psychological, in which case we have an elaborate system of psychiatric nomenclature which we can apply. We rarely describe a person as being lonely and sad; rather, we tend to diagnose him as having a "depression." If a person worries, we say that he has an "anxiety state." And so on. Our basic assumption of disease underlies this drive to diagnose. A diagnosis once made leads to treatment — the final step in the application of the disease model. By treatment we usually mean what we do to the patient — treatment is rarely something the person does for himself, or even something he can do for himself.

The process of medicine — the systematic application of the disease model through examination, diagnosis and treatment — is clearly an excellent system, as far as it goes. It is certainly the best possible way to identify those disease states in which scientific medicine is so helpful. Unfortunately, people have far more symptoms than they do diseases, and the disease model, designed to detect disease, does not always understand and meet the needs of the person. Somewhere around thirty percent of the patients seen in primary care practices in this country have symptoms which are not disease but are expressions through their bodies or moods of some type of human anguish. Frequently these symptoms are somaticized reflections of frustrated needs for personal growth. Problems of the human condition — psychosocial distress, problems of the emotions, the thinking and the spirit of man — affect his body and his total functioning in many ways. Likewise, primary physical disease has important effects on the life and spirit of man.

It is here that one must transcend the disease model in order to fully serve the patient. A wider perspective is needed — what may be called a humanistic, or a growth, model — in which man is seen as a whole and the clinical problem is seen and defined in relation to that whole.

I would like to review three patients who can be seen as examples of what commonly happens in everyday medical practice. The importance of seeing the whole person in relationship to his symptoms will emerge from these cases.

❖   ❖   ❖

RUTH B: (Abstracted from a university medical-center chart)
Age 21; P-0, G-1, LC-0, married; nurses' aide.

Present Illness: Recurrent lower abdominal pain; pelvic pain, mostly right-lower quadrant, of two years' duration with variable vomiting, constipation, weight loss, dysuria, irregular menses, headaches.

Onset: Two months after a normal delivery.

Physical Exam: Negative on most examinations except for tenderness in the RLQ and right pelvis on bimanual pelvic exam, occasionally guarding and rebound are noted.

Lab: Urine, CBC, ESR, vaginal secretions usually negative.

Chronology: (Note: The *chief complaint* in each of these visits is lower abdominal pain.)

4/19 Gyn. Clinic. *Impression* (tentative diagnosis): Cystitis. Rx: Pyridium. Urine culture later reported negative.

6/7   Gyn. Clinic. Constipation and additional symptoms. *Impression:* Colon disease? Hypothyroid? Refer to medical clinic.

6/21   *Emergency Room. Impression:* Anxiety. Rx: Meprobamate. Reassurance.

6/22   Medical Clinic. *Impression:* Lower abdominal pain, etiology undetermined. Rule out chronic pelvic inflammatory disease and urine infection. No evidence of endocrine or G.I. disease; mild anxiety. Urinalysis, BA enema and lumbosacral X-ray negative. Refer to Gyn. Clinic.

6/22   Gyn. Clinic. *Impression:* Pelvic inflammatory disease. Rx: Tetracycline.

7/2   *Emergency Room.* "Can't move legs," an additional symptom. P.E.: Negative. No impression recorded. Return to Gyn. Clinc.

10/8   Gyn. Clinic. Missed period, an additional symptom. *Impression:* Functional irregular uterine bleeding.

10/17   Emergency Room. *Impression:* Twisted right ovarian cyst. Hospitalize for immediate surgery.

10/17   Hospitalized on Gyn. Service. *Impression:* Ovarian cyst with rupture or torsion. Pelvic inflammatory disease. *Surgery:* Culdoscopy, dilatation and curettage, both negative. No ovarian cyst found. Medical consultation (post-op). *Impression:* "Consider porphyria, biliary tract disease, urine infection, allergic vasculitis. It would seem, too, that psychologic factors play a large part." *Psychiatric consultation:* Psychological background described. *Impression:* Psychophysiological reaction. Referral to Psychiatry Clinic recommended. *Discharge diagnosis:* (1) Possible chronic peri-oophoritis, mild; or pelvic inflammatory disease, chronic, mild; (2) Possible acute anxiety reaction. To be followed in Gyn. Clinic.

11/9   Gyn. Clinic. *Impression:* "Acute abdominal pain due to obscure cause." Episode resolved.

March, following year.

Gyn. Clinic. Physical exam and pelvic pneumogram. Small left ovarian cyst; normal right ovary. Rx: Enovid.

4/12   Emergency Room. *Impression:* Ruptured or twisted ovarian cyst. Acute appendicitis. Hospitalize for observation and possible surgery.

4/12   Hospitalized on Gyn. Service. *Impression* (three physicians): Ovarian cyst disease or appendicitis. *Surgery:* Exploratory laparotomy and appendectomy. Pelvic organs normal. No cyst found. Appendix described as "firm"; *Post-op Diagnosis:* Incipient appendicitis. Pathology report: Normal appendix. *Discharge diagnosis:* Pelvic pain, obscure etiology.

8/10   Gyn. Clinic. Several visits, irregular menses. *Impression:* Early pregnancy.

8/22   Hospitalized on Gyn. Service Similar symptoms but febrile. *Admission Impression:* Infected abortion or pelvic inflammatory disease. Dilatation and curettage, negative. No pregnancy found. *Discharge diagnosis:* Gastroenteritis, pseudocyesis.

9/12   Gyn. Clinic. Followup visit. Referred to Medical Clinic. *Impression:* Low abdominal pain, chronic, unknown etiology.

❖❖❖

In Summary (to date of 9/12 medical visit): Illness two years' duration, encompassing twenty visits, three hospitalizations, three surgical procedures, one pelvic pneumogram, four drug therapies, seventeen physicians, sixteen different organic disease diagnoses, and two psychological diagnoses. *Condition:* Unchanged.

❖ ❖

The case history may appear unusually extended and complex, but most physicians will, in reading it, recall that they too have been caught in a similar web of circumstances — a web of multiple organic diagnoses, continued symptomatology, and ineffective drug treatments. Note that during the third visit, on 6/21, a diagnosis of "anxiety" was made; however the patient is not helped in connecting this emotion with her pelvic discomfort. Rather, an attempt is made to block the disagreeable feeling with a tranquilizing drug and reassurance. Additional symptoms appear on 7/2 which further suggest that there is more to Ruth's problem than pelvic disease. Despite this, the struggle to obtain a purely organic diagnosis continues.

During the first hospitalization in October (10/17-10/22), a definitive surgical procedure is done to inspect the pelvic organs, and they are found normal. The attention then shifts to consultation from Internal Medicine and Psychiatry. The internist suggests two rarely-encountered diseases — porphyria and vasculitis. The psychiatrist recognizes that the pain is a reflection and a manifestation of the condition of the patient's life. As may often be the case, this analysis does not satisfy the existing mental set and the recommendation to follow this line of thought is dropped. The chimera of physical disease is pursued, and finally an exploratory laparotomy is carried out. This is an appropriate procedure when there is reasonable doubt about the presence or absence of organic disease. Organic disease is ruled out; the patient remains symptomatic and undiagnosed.

As we noted earlier, many practicing physicians will recognize this situation. Despite our sustained effort, despite numerous trips to the library and multiple consultations, the disease model has failed us in our effort to be of service to our patient. We have all at some time experienced the frustration and resentment of this situation. Paradoxically, it sometimes seems that we, as physicians, are more comfortable diagnosing diseases which we are trained to treat than we are in dealing with human process and human problems.

When Ruth was referred to me, with her extensive medical evaluation, I had little choice but to see her as a healthy person and to look at her symptomatology within the context of her individual life process. My physical examination and lab tests were normal and confirmed this impression. In a series of six interviews between 9/25 and the following January, I explored with her the possible meanings of her pelvic pain. Ruth was quickly able to relate an unhappy marriage and a need for further education to this symptom, and make needed changes in her life. The pain gradually subsided as her life situation became more satisfying to her.

When I think back about this woman and the pelvic pain which plagued her for more than two years, I see her complaints as an expression of conflict and frustrated energy. It is not always possible, of course, for the persons who become patients to be aware of their needs or to make the changes needed, if that is appropriate. When it is possible, a humanistic milieu provides an opportunity for this growth to occur. In the disease model, the patient becomes locked into the system, and as long as diagnosis and treatments are applied, the patient is passive and his attention is diverted from the option for growth. In a humanistic approach, the physician attempts an understanding of the person, and the clinical problem is connected to the human condition. As Dr. Remen has indicated in her case presentation, emphasis is placed on the inner strength of the patient and how the patient can mobilize his own strength in his behalf. Fortunately, as was true with Ruth, there is a great impetus for health in many people which can become manifest if we do not capture them within our system of disease.

The second case I would like to discuss is Evelyn R., a 55-year-old woman, married, who has suffered headaches for ten years. When first seen, Evelyn was taking Codeine (240 mgms daily) and visiting an emergency room on the average of twice monthly for Demerol injections. In preceding years, Evelyn had been seen by many physicians, including a neurologist and other specialists, and numerous special tests had been done. For Evelyn too, the possible value of the disease model had been exhausted: all her studies and examinations were normal, her pains had intensified as more powerful drugs were applied to obliterate them. Her physician referred her to me for consultation, hoping I might suggest additional methods of approaching this difficult situation.

My physical and neurological examinations were also normal. There was nothing that suggested a disease state, and it was not difficult to suspect that her persistent headaches might express some chronic distress in her life. My first approach was to explore her marriage with her and her husband. An extended interview revealed very little. George R. was clearly a loving and devoted husband, and their marriage seemed compatible. They had a nice home, no economic problems, and children who were married, healthy and successful. They were fully cooperative during our talks, and yet no conflict was apparent in their lives. It is possible to respond to this situation by classifying this woman as having an "endogenous or involutional depression" — that is, a depression without apparent conflict or cause. Once this psychiatric diagnosis is made, treatment with mood-elevating drugs is thought appropriate and is usually begun.

However, in man there is a dimension other than conflict which bears consideration. There is in many people the need for purposiveness, for meaning and value, for goals and a future. Sensitivity to this dimension of man is an essential component of a humanistic approach, and sometimes leads to understanding of a clinical problem even when psychoanalytic approaches have failed. Using this perspective, it was easily determined that Evelyn saw her life, though pleasant, as having no purpose. With her children grown, no job, and a self-reliant husband, she had lost her previous identities as mother, homemaker and employee. She had become arrested in her personal development. Life was empty and meaningless.

Her path to health came through encouraging a quest for personal growth in place of the quest for a diagnosis. Evelyn's husband was enlisted as a support in his wife's exploration of her interests. In the enthusiasm and optimism which followed, her headaches improved and narcotics were discontinued.

In the next few months they developed a mutual interest in gardening and a minor hobby of collecting driftwood, into a business involving the manufacture of original and decorative driftwood planters. Evelyn also developed an interest in macrame, and began making rather lovely holders for the planters. They did this together, and, simple as it was, this combination of personal creativity and social usefulness was sufficient to put meaning once again into Evelyn's life.

At present, Evelyn has a little store where she sells planters and meets other people who also love plants. Evelyn and George spend frequent weekends together in Northern California searching for driftwood. She suffers an occasional minor headache when over-tired, but is otherwise quite well and happy.

❖❖❖

Such problems concerning values are very common, and when present may be expressed in physical symptoms. We will not recognize the underlying needs of our patients for values and meanings if we cling to the conventional cause-and-effect model of traditional psychiatry. This approach explores the past and present conflicts, but it does not explore the quest of the person for growth and meaning in life. The patient must become aware of these needs and set forth again on such a path.

The third patient is not an actual person, but a composite of many who represent a common medical problem. This composite is designed to demonstrate some basic differences between the disease and humanistic models, in situations which manifest in physical signs as well as symptoms. The case history and the disease approach to it are outlined in Figure 1.

This patient notices some minor dizzy spells and consults his physician. An examination was negative except for the discovery of hypertension. Operating through the disease model the physician formulates a diagnosis of essential hypertension. The laboratory studies appropriate to this diagnosis were completed. This included a general examination, as well as an investigation of possible organic causes for hypertension. All laboratory tests proved negative — supporting the original diagnosis.

Patient:	Male, age 50
History:	Dizzy spells
Physical Exam:	Negative except BP 150/100
DX:	*Essential hypertension*
Lab:	Routine: CBC, SMA 6/60 and 12/60, urine, EKG, chest X-ray. Special: Hypertensive IVP, 24 hour. Urine for VMA. Sodium, plasma renin.
RX:	*Chlorothiazide B.I.D.*
Following Year:	Six office visits, five electrolyte panels to monitor K+. *RX:* Add KCL, later D.C. Chlorothiazide, add Aldactazide.
Conclusion:	*Patient with chronic disease; hypertension under treatment.*
Results:	Satisfactory; B.P. 130/85

Figure 1.

The patient is now treated with the standard drugs for hypertension. As all drugs have side-effects, treatment necessitates the usual number of follow-up visits and monitoring of the effects of therapy. At the end of a year, both the patient and the physician regard the treatment as successful — the blood pressure is normal.

The Growth Model

Let's take the same hypothetical patient to a physician who uses another approach, attempting to fit the clinical problem together with the human condition of the patient. (See Figure 2.)

This physician sought to understand the problem as a whole. Why the dizzy spells? Although hypertension does occasionally cause dizziness, the presenting blood pressure is not in itself high enough to cause this symptom. Perhaps the dizzy spells and the elevated blood pressure are both reactions to other factors in the patient's life. A few questions are asked, and the doctor listens — a recent business failure, some problems in marriage; resulting tendencies to eat, drink and smoke too much, and not to sleep enough. These are stress factors in this patient's life — factors which could make him feel dizzy at times, as well as produce a reactive hypertension.

This possibility is discussed with the patient, and he is able to understand the meaning of his symptoms within his life. A routine laboratory survey is ordered, including the same analysis of basic organ functions; but the special tests for the unusual organic causes of hypertension are deferred. Such exotic tests may not prove necessary.

During the following year, the patient is able to decide upon and implement changes in his life. His dizzy spells disappear and his blood pressure returns to normal. Two visits document that the blood pressure has returned to normal. No further laboratory tests are necessary, nor are drugs prescribed. At the end of a year, both doctor and patient regard the episode as closed — more importantly, the patient is a normotensive person, *who sees himself as well.* His experience has taught him a great deal about his

Patient:	Male, age 50
History:	Dizzy spells
Physical Exam:	Negative except BP 150/100
DX:	Nervous tension (dizzy spells, labile hypertension)
Lab:	Routine lab only; no special lab tests.
RX:	Discussion of life factors; reduce tobacco and alcohol intake; reduce weight; more sleep.
Following Year:	Two visits, no lab, no drugs.
Conclusion:	Healthy person, BP: 130/55; Reactive hypertension secondary to stress.

Figure 2.

needs and values, and how his body responds to stress — information he has effectively used to care for himself and order his life.

❖❖❖

Both approaches result in normalization of the blood pressure. However, when the disease model is applied strictly, as in the first approach, the patient becomes a normotensive person *who sees himself as sick with a chronic illness,* a reduced life-expectancy, a limited potential, a dependency on doctors and continuing drug therapy. If we put these two approaches side by side in the following chart, we notice a dramatic difference in cost, in addition to the more important ramifications of the self-conception resulting from "chronic illness" on the left, as opposed to health on the right. (See Figure 3.)

Obviously, a person who thinks of himself as chronically ill will place a greater financial burden on himself and the medical system than one who thinks of himself as healthy. We should strongly examine the cost burdens placed on people and the medical system by our tendency as physicians to employ a narrow disease model in our work.

Patient: Male, age 50

History: Dizzy spells

Physical Exam: Negative except BP 150/100

DX:

❖ Essential Hypertension

First Exam:	$ 50
Lab:	206
Drugs:	100
Follow-up Visits:	90
Additional Lab:	52
	$498

Result:

Chronically ill person.

DX:

❖ Nervous tension

First Exam:	$ 50
Lab:	88
Drugs:	0
Follow-up Visits:	30
Additional Lab:	0
	$168

Result:

Well person.

Figure 3.

❖❖❖

In summary, the application of the disease model made without an appreciation of the human condition of the patient may result in the wrong diagnosis, inappropriate diagnostic procedures, ineffective therapy, unnecessary hospitalization, extension of disability, iatrogenic disease, and increased cost. We need to approach patients wholistically, if for no reason other than to practice a truly scientific medicine. If we do not appreciate human needs and the manifold way in which they are expressed in the bodies of our patients, then we tend to correlate signs and symptoms with medical conditions to which, in fact, they may have no relationship. A train of events is set in motion which does not resolve the problem, because it does not fill the real needs of the patient. This is costly in terms of both money, time and suffering.

The following is a *working definition of humanistic care*. Dr. Remen's case, those I have presented, and a number of others in the monograph, *Case Studies and Methods in Humanistic Medical Care* illustrate the central points.

ONE: The patient cannot be seen simply as his disease; neither can the health professional limit his care to medical technology. The full healing potential of their relationship often depends on their interaction as whole human beings, and far exceeds the treatment of disease.

TWO: Every person achieves a unique interdependent relationship of body, mind, emotions and spirit, inseparable from other individuals and society. Illness can best be understood as a disturbance within the dynamic balance of these relationships. Health may be defined as the harmony of the whole, and the work of the health professional as aiding in the re-establishment of a more fully conscious equilibrium within the whole.

THREE: The patient and the health professional are colleagues. Their collaboration activates the latent human and biological resources within the patient for healing. The patient is encouraged to be aware of his choices and to become increasingly responsible for his own health, growth and fulfillment.

FOUR: Illness may provide an opportunity for personal growth. The experience of disease may be used creatively to re-evaluate life goals and values, provide clarity in setting priorities and to mobilize previously untapped strengths. The health professional enables the patient to evolve a positive value from the experience of disease, to maintain identity, and reaffirm his dignity as a person.

FIVE: Illness must be seen in the context of the life span of the individual. Indeed, it may have a unique meaning when seen in reference to the total life of the patient. Physical disease and emotional suffering have an individual message for each patient, yielding information about such personal issues as lifestyle, self-worth and the value of time. The knowledge gained through the understanding of this individual meaning may enable the patient to enrich the quality of his or her life.

This working definition or paradigm may help provide a richer framework in which to approach the challenging privilege of caring for patients. As physicians, we need to be more aware of ourselves, and our own humanity — appreciating ourselves as whole human beings, using fully our own minds, bodies, emotions and spirits, to be there more fully for our patients and to allow our patients to be there more fully for us. We need to seek and apply ways to help our patients become more aware of their strengths and how to use them. Then, we can see ourselves as catalysts, as change-agents — activating latent forces within our patients for their healing and growth.

Chapter IV

Phases In Administration Toward Humanistic Goals

Marguerite Abell Nakles, R.N.

This paper makes the case that entire health care institutions can be transformed through administration but that it is a long process, requiring time, the development of special skills and a humanistic method of administration. Administration for humanistic goals has implications for hospital administrators, hospital personnel and for patients concerned with the dehumanization of large medical institutions.

The art of nursing has its deepest roots in the basic needs of man. The word itself comes from the Latin root *nutrio,* "to nurture" — to evoke the actual from the potential. By definition, then, nursing is a profoundly humanistic undertaking, one that is cognizant of both the uniqueness of the individual and his capacity for growth and healing. However, the technical metamorphosis engaging the world at large and all its institutions has impacted upon and modified this definition. Nursing has become a scientific profession deeply involved with the technical advances of medicine. As a consequence, we are often faced with complex machinery and equipment which occupies our attention and distracts us from some of the original concerns of our profession.

The nursing literature struggles with the issue of technical care vs. professional care, often indicating that these functions may actually require different people — one line of professionals trained to perform the technical skills and one line trained to provide for the individual human needs of the patient.[1]

Though nurses function at different levels of responsibility based on their educational background, to consider that humanness should be the concern of some, while technical skills are the concern of others, is an impossible dichotomy.

It is this very dichotomy which creates frustration and anger in many nurses, especially new graduates who are vividly in touch with the ideals and goals that originally prompted them to choose the profession. Despite these commonly held ideals and goals, it is a fact that patients today frequently charge the system, its nurses and its hospitals, with dehumanized care. "The hospitalized patient is literally an inmate of a total institution, wholly dependent on nurses for care and cut off from the usual sources of information and social support needed to assume an active role in making decisions."[2] Indeed, the dehumanization process in hospitals is often quite complete. We place the patient in the vertical position, replace clothes with a white, often wrinkled shirt that never seems to cover the right places at the right time, attach an unremovable name tag and number to a wrist, assume full responsibility for bowels, sleep, and food habits, and take away the personal sense of day and night. A patient's former identity as a self-determining adult may be replaced by that of a dependent, passive, helpless, non-being.

Obviously, none of us means to create this result. It derives, rather, from a complex system attempting to give responsible, high quality professional care. But if we are to answer legitimate complaints, we need to begin by squarely facing such problems. This loss of individual dignity is a needlessly high price to pay for hospital care. Furthermore, people are generally beginning to defend their dignity and humanness: members of our society are becoming outspokenly critical, demanding to participate in their care rather than just be cared for by their institutions. Therefore, an unresponsive, or worse, dictatorial attitude on the part of nurses and hospitals is increasingly likely to cause society as a whole to actively attempt to alter the medical system.

However, the system itself can respond positively and creatively to the challenges of new conditions. The history of nursing indicates that the profession has generally been both responsive to changing social conditions and also actively responsible for changing them. The more than 1,300,000 American nurses, active and inactive, currently and formerly licensed, represent the largest body of health personnel educated and equipped to perform at a critical level of skill.[3] They represent, therefore, an enormous potential for effecting a real advance in health care delivery. They are a great resource for furthering the goals of humanistic patient care.

Developing Humanistic Institutions
Through Nursing Administration

Our present society has become sufficiently dehumanized that people often stand alone and separated even in times of illness and stress. Nurses and hospitals need to know how to respond to these and similar needs of the ill in society today, including needs for caring, maintenance of self-respect, recognition and enhancement of individuality, and the development of purpose and meaning. In general, traditional nursing education has not fully prepared nurses to respond to such needs of the patient, and traditional hospital institutions have not been developed around these goals. The challenge in nursing administration is to evoke this latent human potential within existing institutions and then provide the education and the practical framework for the implementation of humanistic care.

History and many present indicators would lead to the belief that nursing and nurses will ultimately be able to respond creatively to the human needs of their patients in appropriate new ways. As a first step, I believe that responsibility must be accepted for creating an environment, a *climate of willingness* for health professionals to be trained in and to practice humanistic care. I hoped to develop such an environment four years ago when I accepted my position as Vice President and Director of Nursing at Marshal Hale Hospital in San Francisco. Marshal Hale is a 150 bed general hospital staffed by approximately 250 registered nurses, licensed vocational nurses and nurses' aides. Part of my job responsibility involves the setting of standards and quality of nursing care and the overall administration of the Nursing Department. In 1971, Marshal Hale Memorial Hospital was a good general hospital with all the strengths and all the shortcomings of contemporary technological institutions. Creating an environment favorable to the evolution of humanistic professional care, within such an institution, is a gradual process.

At the present stage of analysis four phases have emerged as necessary to developing humanistic hospital care: *creating readiness in the nursing staff and the institution; developing basic tools and methods for teaching humanistic nursing; devising and conducting in-service training curricula; and finally, implementing the application of humanistic principles and methods in clinical nursing care through changes in physical and organizational structure.* The first phase has already been implemented at Marshal Hale and is described below. The plans for the next phases are also described.

Phase One:
The Development of "Readiness"

Bringing staff nurses to the point where they feel and express the desire to have a supportive, nurturing relationship with the patient takes time, commitment and skills. The methods I have found most effective are *focusing* staff attention on humanistic concerns and *modeling* humanistic attitudes and behavior. I began by personally getting to know the staff, attempting to model in this process the kinds of attitudes and behaviors needed. Accordingly, I was interested in knowing not just their ages and where they were educated, but their hopes, aspirations and goals. I initiated a program of personal conversations and have spoken with many of the nurses on the staff.

One of my goals for this phase has been to help nurses rediscover and re-experience that part in them who had chosen a life of service — the reasons why they originally entered the profession. All too frequently the early devotion and caring so prevalent among student nurses turns to frustration, cynicism, and hostility as unprepared nurses try vainly to implement their sincere desires to be humanistic in an environment of high pressure, short-staffed units, and acutely ill and dying patients. Hearing, in these conversations, the personal and deeply humanistic ideals of the staff was frequently an enriching and enlightening experience both for me and for the individual staff person. These conversations convinced me to pursue my goal of developing a humanistic hospital in order to enable the full expression of these ideals. I have shared my own ideals with the staff and used the opportunity to focus each nurse on her role as a model and teacher of human caring and health to patients and other health personnel alike. I feel now that I know the staff and have modeled to them my personal ability and willingness to see each of them, not only as a colleague but also as a full person.

Two of these interviews come to mind as typical of the work during this first phase of creating readiness. During my hospital rounds, I had witnessed several instances of angry behavior and generalized discontent in one of the staff nurses. Marion was described by her supervisors as "very unhappy and annoyed." When I questioned her about her anger, she expressed dissatisfaction with staffing procedures, job performance by her aides, and "things in general." She told me she had been out of college and licensed just six months; I was surprised, because new graduates are usually enthusiastic and idealistic. During our conversation I decided to pursue her dissatisfactions to whatever end they might take us. I soon discovered that just beneath her negativity lay a tremendous caring and devotion. She began to cry as she expressed frustration and resentment at not having time to provide individual and supportive care for her patients. She described the conflict between her vision of ideal nursing and what she found in the real world of the hospital. She felt she barely had time to complete the tasks required by the patient's physical condition and could rarely spend additional time to care for them as individuals. I, too, had experienced this pressure on many occasions and told her so. I explained that I dealt with the conflict of time in terms of human quality. The amount of time spent is not the real issue: it is the human quality of time, as measured by the message received by the patient, that is the important thing. The task is to deliver the message: "I care for you as a person and I accept who you are." This message can often be quickly communicated by a brief gentle touch, or by a passing warmth in voice and manner. I described my dream of a humanistic hospital and we shared our common belief in the importance of such values and ideals.

Marion said she had not known who I really was and had never considered what my goals might be. She left my office expressing a desire to deal with the hard business of a busy nursing unit and still provide humanistic care. Rather than seeing her as a malcontent, I now knew that we shared a similar vision. I planned to include Marion in the inservice training that would be part of phase three.

Not long after my conversation with Marion, another nurse, Barbara, requested that I stop and see a patient on her unit when I made rounds. This patient had been admitted for depression and Barbara thought he was possibly suicidal. She reported she felt unable to "make him better" and was depressed by her inability to discharge this heavy responsibility.

We visited the patient, Arthur W. together. Arthur's depression appeared to have been precipitated by his wife's suing him for divorce. He apologized for crying, but talked of suicide and said that he felt he was "too weak to live without her." After listening carefully, I told him that I trusted his sadness and tears, but not his weakness. I suggested that he focus on his strength, which, of course he denied having. I told him that he might try *acting as if* he had strengths and suggested that he write those strengths down. "Acting as if" and the writing down of psychological insights are useful techniques in personal growth.[4]

The next day Barbara called my office. Arthur had asked that we come to see him again as soon as possible. When we arrived, he showed us what he had written — three pages, on both sides, all about his strengths and how he had been giving away his power to his wife. "Quite a lot of strength to develop overnight," he said with pride. He seemed less depressed and expressed positive feelings. He left the hospital the following day under the care of a psychiatrist. He told us that he planned to continue writing about his feelings and thoughts, his present life and his future.

Barbara and I discussed this patient in terms of responsibility and choice. Her feeling that *she* was responsible to make him better had been unrealistic and unnecessary. Arthur, like most of us, has a great deal of strength of which he was largely unaware. He had to be helped to mobilize his *own* inner strength and then to take responsibility for helping himself. She expressed great relief, as she had never thought in terms of patients having the strength to choose and be more responsible for themselves. In my work as a nurse, I too had been burdened by my belief that I was totally responsible for the life of a patient. We shared our mutual satisfaction at being able to collaborate and share responsibility with the patient.

This interview and the preceding one are examples of modeling humanistic attitudes, in order to more systematically focus staff attention to the needs of the whole person who is the patient. Still another approach in the initial phase is to meet in unit groups with nursing staff every month. These meetings give us an opportunity to share appreciation and resentments concretely — and to collectively experience our common goals and ideals. After eight months of these group meetings, the staff has begun to request additional training for achieving more humanistic nursing care. They have also begun suggesting other changes aimed towards the furthering of this goal. Sensing the readiness to accept change, I have begun reorganizing the nursing assignments in each unit of the hospital, enabling a nurse to continue caring, as much as possible, for the same patients whenever she works. Each patient now has contact with a maximum of five or six nurses rather than ten or twelve, as in the previous system. In our unit meetings we discuss implementing other structural changes along the same lines. An atmosphere of readiness has been achieved and phase one is nearing completion.

The second and third phases in building a humanistic hospital are the development of tools for teaching humanistic nursing and the design and conduct of humanistic nursing curricula. Borrowing on educational tools developed in such fields as humanistic psychology and confluent education, a teaching model has been developed for inservice training in humanistic concepts and methods, which I hope to implement during the coming year.[5]

The focus of the teaching model will be on the person as an integrated complex of body, mind, feelings, will, and spirit.[6] Each participant will have the opportunity to personally explore these human aspects and then to begin integrating their discoveries into their personal and professional lives. This expanded view of the person opens possibilities for the nursing practitioner to expand the dimensions of nursing care. In response to an awareness of the full potential of nursing and the growing need to begin to implement this potential, specific methods will be presented and examined. Such methods may include non-verbal communication, responsibility training, biofeedback, and journal writing, among many others.

Simultaneously with the second and third phases, the fourth phase, that of creating the concrete physical and organizational structure to accommodate humanistic care, must begin. Such administrative decisions as the reorganization of nursing assignments referred to on page 62 are a part of the fourth phase, and create institutional forms to assist nurses wishing to synthesize new values into their roles as skilled practitioners.

Marshal Hale is at the beginning of a long and slow process, but the message is becoming clear — a humanistic hospital can be developed within the existing system, despite the usual emergencies, time pressures, staffing difficulties, and budgetary constraints. Such a hospital provides for the education and involvement of all people who work there. The changes in attitudes and the interest in implementing humanistic goals expressed by the nursing staff have evoked the interest of other Departments within the hospital. At the request of the Vice President of Finance, and of the personnel of the Admitting Department and the Financial Department, I will be meeting with them to discuss our common goals of care. Out of these discussions may come an eagerness and a program for other hospital workers to participate in the delivery of humanistic care in their daily encounters with patients and their families.

❖❖❖

The slowness of this process must be emphasized. In my own enthusiasm and out of my conviction, my first inclination was to rush in, call a general meeting, explain what humanistic care was about, and then to insist that all staff members embark on a personal development program to prepare themselves for their new role. Obviously, this would have been improper, unwise and futile. Administratively, values cannot be imposed from outside, they must be evoked from within.

Making the potential of a hospital like Marshal Hale into an actuality requires not authority but the essential ingredient of nursing — nurture. All the dimensions of humanistic nursing are already present in the existing health care system. The move requires not revolution, but evolution through a synthesis of technical scientific skills with a humanly sensitive staff and environment.

Chapter V

Professional Education
for
Humanistic Medicine

Sara Unobskey Miller, M.A.

This paper concerns the critical dimension of professional training for humanistic goals and draws attention to underlying principles of humanistic health professional education. Focusing on such general principles is vital if educational efforts toward humanism are not to lose themselves in absorption with particular techniques.

To achieve a new medicine which is both scientifically effective and humanly relevant, we must first acknowledge that medicine as an institution does not exist apart from its individual practitioners. The humanistic evolution of contemporary medicine is not possible without a parallel evolution of the individual practitioner. Therefore, we need to conceive and implement a professional education that seriously and systematically attempts the achievement of humanistic goals.

Such humanistic training cannot be based simply on training in alternative medical techniques, no matter how much they may appear to offer ways of implementing humanistic values in medical practice. For example, the methods outlined in our own early monograph, *Case Studies and Methods in Humanistic Medical Care*, are not an adequate basis for humanistic practice. They, and some of the intriguing methodologies we have heard discussed at this conference — like biofeedback, acupuncture and inner imagery — are only methodologies. They may eventually, perhaps, be some of the tools of humanistic medicine, as existing medicine has important tools of surgery, x-ray and laboratory diagnosis. But methodologies will only be humanistic if the person using the method is himself humanistic; such a person will be able to use any methodology toward humanistic purposes. The establishment of a humanistic medicine depends, then, on evoking and nourishing certain qualities and awarenesses in the medical practitioner, qualities which inform the use of all of his techniques, both traditional and non-traditional. Without these awarenesses the practitioner — no matter how enlightened his methods — is merely another technician.

I have had principal responsibility for developing an educational program that we hoped would provide a basis for humanistic innovations in medical thinking and practice. In three years of work with a group of traditionally educated and highly successful medical practitioners, several important patterns of conceptual change and individual evolution emerged. The commonality of these patterns of re-education leads me to suspect that a similar process may be generally essential to the education of other health professionals interested in achieving a personal basis for humanistic practice. These patterns can be formulated as preliminary principles of humanistic medical training. I do not mean to suggest these are the only principles, but I believe they provide a good point of departure for further work. In our experience the following issues underlie the evolution of the professional from a highly trained and effective contemporary health professional to a highly trained and effective contemporary humanistic health professional:

1. An expanded conceptual understanding of the personality structure of the individual.

2. An expanded view of time.

3. A deeper understanding of the relationship between disease and illness.

4. An expanded view of the nature of pain.

5. An expanded view of the role of the health professional.

These issues were not taken up in any particular order or sequence in our training program. Rather all these issues were often dealt with simultaneously. We have found that there is no one way to teach the necessary expansion of ideas and concepts. The actual learning experiences that will create such educational outcomes are varied and can be drawn, as we have done, from a multitude of sources, such as philosophy, psychology, psychophysiology, sociology, religion, anthropology, systems theory, literature and the arts. The issues in themselves then might be thought of as the basis of a "core curriculum" in the education of the professional — each teacher and each student dealing with the issues in his own individual way.

❖❖❖

Let me briefly discuss each of these essential issues:

1. *An expanded conceptual understanding of the personality structure of the individual.*
If a health professional is to practice a new medicine — a medicine based on the full nature of man — his view of the nature of man must indeed be a full one — realistic and accurate. Our view of the person both determines and limits the breadth of care we give. If the patient is seen as essentially a body, the health professional will tend to direct therapeutic efforts to the body alone. If the patient

is largely seen as a body with a mind, the health professional may seek to help the patient toward a cognitive clarity about the disease in addition to conventional diagnosis and treatment. Finally, if the patient is seen as a body with feelings, the health professional may use a psychosomatic approach.

All three of these aspects of the person can be synthesized, in which case we get a rich result, allowing for flexible appreciation of the patient along these three dimensions, singly and in combination. This view of the patient may be diagrammed as follows:

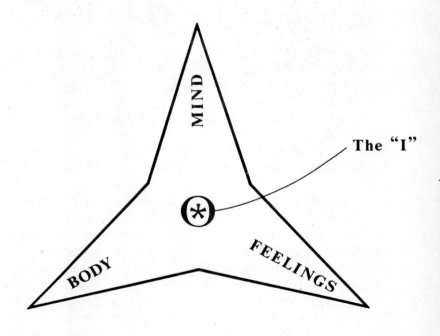

Figure   1

But this is only a step to a fuller understanding. We have found that humanistic care requires a view of the personality and consciousness which takes into account not only the patient's body, feelings and mind, but such other attributes as values, higher creativity and will. This more inclusive view of the personality is expressed in Figure 2.[1]

The Freudian or "lower" unconscious indicated in the diagram, the source of our atavistic and biological drives, is well-known in medicine. In addition to an understanding of this level of man, health professionals need a complementary understanding of the "higher" unconscious or superconscious. This can be described as the autonomous realm from which orginate our more highly evolved impulses, including humanitarian action, artistic and scientific inspiration, philosophic and spiritual insight, and the impulse for purpose and meaning in life. No accurate view of the patient can exclude an awareness of this level of human nature and its multiple effect on the body, feelings, mind and their dynamic interrelationships. Figure 2 also places the will in a central position — the will being the capacity to choose and change. The will is a force which is gradually being recognized as a major factor in the maintenance of health and the recovery from illness. The "will-to-live" has been recognized as a factor in mortality since the time of Hippocrates. But only now are we beginning to envision the possibility of engaging the patient's will systematically and deliberately as a routine step in restoring and maintaining health.

Figure 2 also includes a transpersonal or "higher self," an inner source of wisdom and guidance. It has been described as "the part which knows."[2] Many of us have intuitive wisdom about our needs and our own direction.

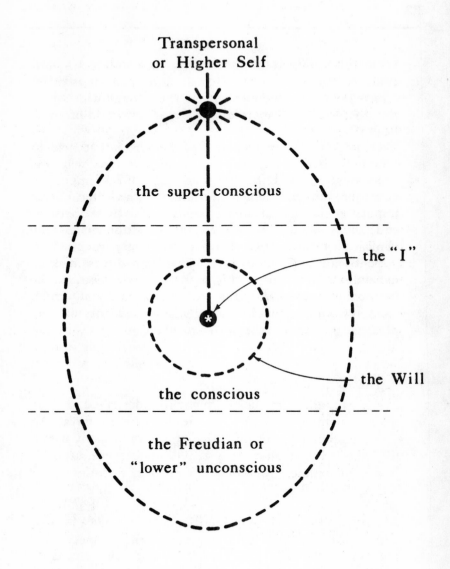

Transpersonal
or Higher Self

the super conscious

the "I"

the conscious

the Will

the Freudian or
"lower" unconscious

Figure 2

Within the context of medicine such a higher self may come to function as Dr. Remen noted, as an auxiliary "inner doctor" — a dimension of the patient with which the doctor can collaborate in a mutual effort to promote health.

Operating from an awareness of the person that includes not only body, feelings and mind but also will, the superconscious and the transpersonal self has important consequences for medicine, some of which have been implied in the clinical cases presented by both Dr. Barbour and Dr. Remen. The professional's assessment of the clinical problem may be changed and his assessment of the patient's inner resources for dealing with disease may be expanded. In addition, this more inclusive view of the personality also enriches the professional's view of himself and, accordingly, he can bring many more of his own personal resources to the professional encounter.

2. An expanded view of time.

Contemporary medicine might be described as the science of the effective use of the short time interval. An understanding of brief time quanta and their many uses is well-taught by the current system of medical education. It is not uncommon for complete medical histories to be taken, disease diagnosed and alleviated and even lives saved all within the fifteen minute interval of the traditional office visit. However, few practitioners have been educated with equal sensitivity to a long range time perspective — that sense of time which goes beyond the immediate health intervention. Even when the health professional does adopt a longer perspective, he often proceeds in a narrowly confined manner, adopting, for example, the time frame dictated by a chronic or terminal disease. Thus, it is the chronology of the disease which dominates and not the time dimension of the life of the patient who is the raison d'etre of the health care interaction. It has been our experience that traditionally educated health professionals rarely see their work with, for example, a twenty year old patient who is not chronically ill, as a part of a fifty year program of health maintenance and promotion. This limited time perspective and its implications are not an adequate basis for humanistic care.

The patient has a relationship to his own body, and to his own health which endures for more than a quarter of an hour. The patient also has a relationship to the health care system which is life long and far exceeds the duration of relationship to any individual practitioner. What is experienced during a brief office visit may, therefore, have an effect on the content and quality of health over a patient's lifetime and must be seen in such a perspective. Once the health professional achieves an expanded sense of time, the individual visit can be seen in this perspective and the opportunity can be effectively used — promotively and preventively. As a matter of usual contemporary practice, however, the goal is generally short range — to resolve the partient's immediate problem. The educational dimension of the interaction is often overlooked.

It has been our experience that a *personal* understanding of the time dimensions in which individual human beings and groups. actually live, is critical if the health professional is to begin to see his patients in an extended time frame. Practitioners need to experience their own lives as a *process,* in order to recognize the lives of others as a process as well. Such experience importantly changes the view of many of the fundamentals of medicine; for example, the realization that illness may, in some cases, over the long range, and with appropriate support, positively influence the quality of an individual's life.[3] The direction of human process can be profoundly changed by impact at a single point. The fifteen minute office visit may represent such an opportunity; an awareness of this possibility makes such a meaningful exchange more likely.

3. A deeper understanding of the relationship between disease and illness.

Disease is the pathology which the doctor diagnoses from the problems the patient presents to him. In contrast, "illness" indicates the personal experience of disease and takes into account the entire person, including, his attitudes, feelings, thoughts, and values that surround, reflect and indeed often define his disease.

Within the limitations of the disease concept, all patients with diabetes are essentially the same. Within the concept of illness each is different: the experience has a unique meaning and a unique effect on the total life process of each patient. The physician trained in contemporary western medicine is often an expert on disease but frequently not knowledgeable about illness. He may practice within a limited model of disease and health, a truly mechanistic view of body parts which have broken down and must be repaired. Within this construct there is little role for the patient except to notify the health repair system when a part is not functioning; the health professional bears then the main responsibility for effecting change.

By contrast the concept of illness intimately involves the patient. who alone is privy to internal process: only the patient truly knows his own thoughts, feelings, concerns and values. Unlike the "replace-or-repair" modality derived from the disease concept, the illness concept recognizes that the patient, with his potential for effecting wholistic change, must be central to the medical enterprise. While the physician may prescribe specific therapy for the body, only the patient can go on to actually integrate the experience of disease and heal his life. From such a perspective, there is indeed, a "healthy way to have a disease."[4] The physician who sees his patients as people with illness — an experience rich with implications — is in a position to allow and facilitate the process of patient growth and to begin to practice a fully humanistic medicine.

4. An expanded view of pain.

The concept of illness allows that a disease is potentially an educative experience, a stimulus or catalyst for the patient and his physician. The same is true of an expanded understanding of the major symptom of disease — pain.

Both the patient and professional share a view of pain which conforms to that of contemporary society: pain is the enemy a totally negative experience to be deplored and avoided. But the issue is not this simple. Literature, religion and ordinary experience teach that the experience of pain can yield valuable information, information about the self and the world. Pain is the common human experience, the great leveler, and can therefore be a powerful tool for breaking down perceived barriers and differences between the self and others. Through the experience of pain we may become acutely aware of our similarity to others, an awareness which may evoke true empathy and compassion. Pain may also lead to a dependence on others that can be quite profound. Consequently, a significant experience of pain may be the first in which an adult does not perceive himself as being fully in control of the outer circumstances of his life situation. This enforced dependency may clarify the nature, meaning and value of all our human relationships, leading to a more accurate notion of human interdependence. Paradoxically, the ordeal of pain and its resolution, may also lead a person to a greater awareness of his individuality and strength. Pain may also force a realistic "intimation of mortality," throwing into illuminating relief such issues as choice of life style, direction, goals and purpose and leading to a re-evaluation of these choices in the patient's life.

Pain can present itself in a number of ways as a teacher: the manner in which it is received will partly determine whether it functions in this way or not. Consequently, it is important that the health professional be aware that, once alleviated, pain can be reflected upon as an experience and provide an opportunity for personal and social understanding. Without this awareness of the value of pain, the patient's experience of pain can be wasted and meaningless.

5. *An expanded view of the role of the health professional.*

It has been our experience that the average health professional is trained both to see himself and to act as a highly competent but obedient soldier in the ranks of the health care system. He or she is trained to take orders and give orders quickly and efficiently. Despite protestations of their individuality, professionals typically do accept a number of largely unquestioned authorities, for instance, the authority of certain journals, certain major or local institutions, certain commanding reputations, the authority of boards of accreditation and licensure, and so forth.

Certainly much of this is necessary, for the collective wisdom of the profession must ensure responsible standards of practice. Unfortunately, however, there are also tremendous defects inherent in the present authoritarian tendency. Too few health professionals see themselves as potential leaders or innovators. All too frequently they see themselves merely as competitors in the struggle to meet a common standard — a standard both established and enforced by others. Consequently, the struggle for intellectual courage and real excellence gets short shrift. The physician's view of himself is not that of a teacher.

The physician's limited view of himself and his role is often expressed when he or she dispenses health as a product rather than models it as a personal process. The profession even seems to disdain and fear itself as anyone who has tried to persuade a doctor to see a doctor will testify. It may be that personal illness is seen by many doctors as equivalent to weakness. The oath of service is indeed deeply instilled and the physician who falls ill may feel that he has betrayed his pledge. The myth of service requires self-sacrifice and illness may be seen as a shameful indication of unfitness for the profession. On the other hand, the notion that the health professional is himself a positive resource of society — to be carefully nurtured and conserved — is not adequately taught. Long and superhuman working hours rather than a realistic conservation and cultivation of personal health are the standard which indicates devotion to service. Their diminished life-expectancy as a group reflects the fact that few medical professionals take sufficient responsibility for their own health. How difficult, then for them to persuasively demand such responsibility from their patients.

But the humanistic health care can not exclude the health professional from its scope. To practice a humanistic medicine a professional must be cultivating personal health in the fullest sense. He must come to see his developing, evolving health, as a part of the contribution that he makes to medicine. This experience then can be modelled and taught.

This aspect of humanistic education — of moving the professional self-concept from that of a technological soldier to a humanistic health model — is perhaps the longest and most subtle of the phases of training. It comes about as a result of a gradual and progressively enriched personal understanding of the concepts discussed under our previous four points. When reached, this stage frequently results in a revitalized interest in practice and also in a greater sense of life.

❖❖❖

In closing, then, let me restate the major premise: the creation of a humanistic medical practice requires education toward humanistic goals. The actual teaching methodologies used to develop personal knowledge of the principles outlined here, will vary according to the student, the teacher, their training situation, and other circumstances in which they find themselves. Vast educational resources already exist both for the cognitive and affective dimensions of education. In many instances, new methodologies must be devised to achieve these profound educational goals. It has been our experience, however, that these goals can be reached and the process of reaching them is a creative and rewarding one.

Chapter VI

Some Principles of a
Health Policy for the Future

Dale Garell, M.D.

This paper surveys the broad but fragmentary national effort already underway to achieve humanistic goals in health care. The four principles suggested for a health policy of the future bring into focus the vital dimension of policy and planning. These principles may be useful in finding solutions to a number of pressing health system problems, including costs, science policy, and the critical issue of what is health.

I think it fair to say that, until quite recently, the general form or paradigm of modern medicine has been remarkably stable. This form has had as one of its major foundations, the disease model — a model which, as Dr. Barbour has said, rather narrowly defines the roles of doctor and patient and the nature of their interaction. The paradigm of modern medicine has also tended to base itself on a mechanistic modality and world view imitating,[1] oddly enough, not the energy physics of our modern day, but rather, the Newtonian physics on which Victorian science was built. Operating within such an approach, many practitioners report it difficult to avoid seeing individual patients as interchangeable. Man tends to be seen as a machine and the health professional, a biological repair man — outfitted with scientific tools.

In recent years, however, there has been a growing set of movements attempting to broaden and enrich the existing medical paradigm. These movements begin from and are possible because of the very successes of modern scientific medicine. The benefits of modern care are increasingly apparent and taken for granted and the flaws, therefore, become more glaring and objectionable. As Dr. Miller has pointed out, a principal problem of modern culture is the dehumanization of science and technology. The major flaw of modern medicine is the dehumanization which results from its paradigm. Accordingly, it is not surprising to find that most of the movements to broaden the paradigm of modern medicine are essentially attempts to remedy the problems of dehumanization in health care.

These efforts at a solution start typically from small beginnings, and then spread to become larger and larger aspects of the established medical scene. They have stirred considerable hope, energy, and enthusiasm from many different constituencies. Collectively, they have tended to increase public and professional consciousness of the larger issues of dehumanization. Individually, they have gone a partial distance toward alleviating the problems. Reviewing these attempts will help us, therefore, to see what further general principles of health policy are necessary if we are to move forward systematically and achieve the synthesis of scientific medicine with humanistic values. These approaches to humanistic medicine include:

The ethical-philosophical approach. This attempt, well exemplified in such institutions as the Hastings Center and the Kennedy Institute, arises in response to the ethical dilemmas inherent in scientific medicine and increasingly faced by health professionals and health policy makers and planners. The insights generated by this particular theoretical approach are needed by clinical practitioners, and the eventual translation of this information into everyday practice will greatly benefit health care.

Movements to rehumanize critical life events. These movements focus on major life events — such as birth, sex, death, and aging — which have dramatically suffered at the hands of modern, highly-organized, highly-technologized medicine. The work of such professionals as Kubler-Ross,

Lenore Schwartz and Gay Luce are some important examples of this approach. For many practitioners, work on such specific problems has created an awareness of and a means of entry into the larger concerns of humanistic medicine.

The humane letters approach. This effort is exemplified by a variety of groups and institutions — such as the Institutes of the Society for Health and Human Values — seeking to introduce instruction in the traditional humanities into medical school curricula or preprofessional education. Exposure to such theoretical, intellectual, and cultural background often creates a willingness and a readiness which enables professional school graduates to seek or develop more humanistic methods of practice.

The behavioral sciences approach. This is another wide-ranging approach, at both pre-professional and professional levels. One main branch parallels the humane letters effort, offering the student cultural background in such disciplines as sociology, psychology and anthropology. Another main branch involves the use of instrumentalities like group dynamics in order to increase communication between practitioners and patients. The work of Human Dimensions in Medical Education at the Center for Studies of the Person is an example of this. In general, the behavioral sciences approach has contributed much to the background health practitioners bring to their encounters with patients. It has also contributed toward better methods and habits of communication, and been useful in facilitating the practitioner's attempt to express caring in his or her own practice.

Alternate therapies. Many of these attempt to enlarge the conceptual paradigm and the general model of medical practice. Biofeedback may be taken as an example. The attempt here has been to reintroduce into medicine the key notion that the patient can be more responsible for his or her own health. Biofeedback and the other alternate therapies can, of course, be reduced in practice simply to *other* therapies, and be applied in the same depersonalized ways that were the sources of the original complaints about dehumanization. But when the fresh perspectives introduced by some of the new therapies are maintained, they help to create an atmosphere of openness in which humanistic agendas can be implemented.

The health team approach. Arising out of the twin needs to reduce costs and to pay medical attention to the whole person this approach stresses the importance of a multidisciplinary effort toward health care. It is exemplified by the work of such institutions as the Institute for Health Team Development. The applications of multidisciplinary perspectives to the problems of dehumanization promises important results for practice and health.

Consumer self-help approaches. Consumer activity, including publications and efforts to devise alternative health care delivery systems, is on the rise. Books suggesting alternatives to high technology medicine are eagerly read by the public resulting in an increasing tendency to foster the creation of self-care modalities for consumers. Specific examples of such self-care modalities include Weight Watchers, drug abuse centers and Alcoholics Anonymous.

These widespread approaches indicate the existence of a large-scale effort to find richer and more personalized ways of conceiving and delivering care. It must be stressed, however, that these efforts, impressive as they are, are distinctly partial and beginning attempts to find a solution to the total problem. What is really needed is the sort of broad innovative thinking which will reconceive the underlying paradigm of contemporary medicine.

❖❖❖

Towards a Humanistic Health Policy

To support the needed broad thinking, as well as the practical and proper evolution of the many approaches already in progress, we should begin to reconceive the postulates and priorities of health policy. Reconceiving health policy in such a light is a large task, one requiring the cooperation of many experts. There are, however, four principles which can, I think, be discussed already, if only in outline form.

1. Health Policy needs to acknowledge that medicine is evolving. Our brief survey of some of the approaches to problems of dehumanization reminds us that medicine is in a continuous process of change. Evolution is a fact of life, a fact of medical life, and a fact which we need to welcome. Fifty years from now, I am reasonably sure, there will be a health care system, but it will be a different system and it should be. This new system will be produced by changes in technology, in society, in the problems the system is asked to address, and so forth. To meet such changing circumstances, *health policy needs to encourage a continuing pluralism* that will ensure appropriate additions to the theory, skill and technology of modern medicine. Promising new technologies, such as many of those discussed at this conference, need full clinical trials. We need to reserve medical judgement and to prepare to be flexible in our acceptance of new tools that prove effective. Likewise, we must be prepared to encourage systematic study of many of the non-technological efforts at humanistic medicine listed above, searching for common premises, evaluating their results, and synthesizing their discoveries. One specific recommendation for health policy that will make this first principle effective is this: the National Health Insurance that is coming must take into account new developments and allow room for their further evolution. In short, for the health of medicine and the health of us all, we must studiously avoid a policy that freezes the medical system into its existing paradigm.

2. Health policy needs to acknowledge the patient as an untapped health resource. The national self-care movements we have alluded to and the observations of Dr. Barbour and others point toward an important possibility: it may be possible to forsee a system of medicine in which the patient is a primary health care provider. Health policy must seriously allow for this real possibility. Dr. Remen has reminded us that health care cannot be successful unless the patient, at one level or another, collaborates with the professional. There is mounting evidence that patients want to assume increasing responsibility for their own care and that they can learn to do so. Other factors compel attention to a policy of patient activation in care: as is well-known, many of the common problems confronting today's medicine are social problems, psychosomatic ills, reactions to physical illness. It is obvious that one person well-situated to take care of such problems of social living is the patient himself. A health policy exploring a participatory approach must allow for the development in health professional education of "consultant" skills. Professionals will need to know how to function in collaboration with the patient, fostering the skills and attitudes necessary to mobilize the patient's inherent ability for active participation. Policy moving in this direction need not reject the valuable technology or the sophisticated skills available to the contemporary health professional. Rather, it will acknowledge that much basic health care can and ought to be delivered directly by the patient.

3. *Health policy needs to support the scientific exploration of man as a unique species.* Medicine has rightly tended to acknowledge the commonality of biological life. However, a human medicine, not to speak of a humanistic medicine, must also give the most serious research attention to man as a unique species. For example, the trend toward the activation of the patient we have described, points toward a crucial human attribute which demands a more systematic scientific investigation: man can choose. We need to understand more about the human will, how it works, and what its impact can be in medicine. Out of such research effort could well come important consequences for the costs, structure and human quality of care. Other uniquely human dimensions — like man's capacity for creating meaning and for affirming values — need similar scientific study of their nature and their relevance to the promotion and re-establishment of health.

4. Health policy needs to promote a deeper understanding of the process of health and to encourage rational action based on that understanding. Health policy needs to promote a deeper understanding of the process of health. We are beginning to recognize for example, that illness is often induced by stress. Even more interesting, we are beginning to know that stress is a normal part of life — that people *need* certain life crises in order to maintain their growth as persons. Such life crises represent a transition, an evolution from one phase of life to another. The absence of crises is in many cases the absence from living. If this is so, we can well understand what many private practitioners report: illness, while unplanned, often seems to fit into the life process of the individual. When a person becomes ill, he is entitled to the time and privacy to think and plan, he has an opportunity to assess values and goals and ways of dealing with stresses. Consciously or unconsciously, he may use the opportunity to retreat and to work on his growth as a person. This is intrinsically a healthy process, a process of health, but it is often below awareness and paradoxically carried on in the context of disease and the sick role.

Emphasizing the health process can have important consequences for health and growth as well as for our institutional life. By paying too exclusive an attention to illness, for example, our society has created a situation in which illness may often be the only acceptable way out of our daily life routines. Yearly, we spend millions, perhaps billions of dollars, reinforcing illness behavior. What would happen however, if industry, for example, would reverse its present tendency to encourage illness instead of encouraging health and growth? What would happen if companies would acknowledge "healthing" behavior, to use Dr. Hoke's phrase, by granting "well leaves" as an alternative to "sick leaves" each year? Would such a reversal of emphasis cut down on unplanned illness and its impact on productivity? Would it increase the person's strength to deal creatively with stress? These are important questions, typical of the new ones we need to ask about the health process.

The creation of a humanistic health policy requires, as I have noted, development and examination of these four principles and others which are being suggested by large events already in motion. The new synthesis of medicine and humanism which has been discussed is going to be achieved only after a long, complex, and cooperative effort by many people — health professionals being only some of these. Health policy has a critical role to play in creatively supporting the emergence of the future medicine. Someone defined a plan as "the intelligent cooperation with the inevitable." I hope that health policy will move in the kinds of directions we have indicated and that the inevitable with which we can all cooperate will be a more humanly relevant and scientific medicine.

NOTES

Chapter I

[1] Quoted in Lawrence LaShan, *The Medium, The Mystic, and the Physicist*, New York, 1974, p. 272. See also the useful appendix in the book, "Physicists and Mystics," which catalogs some additional fifty parallel statements about the nature of reality by eminent physicists and spiritual leaders.

[2] See, for example, George I. Brown, *Human Teaching for Human Learning*, New York, 1971. George I. Brown, Thomas Yeomans and Liles Grizzard (Eds.), *The Live Classroom*, New York, 1975.

[3] For more detailed description of the working process of the original Institute staff, see Stuart Miller, "A New Humanism in Medicine," in SYNTHESIS, Volume 1, Number 1, Spring, 1974, pp. 63-71.

[4] Edmund Pellegrino, "Humanism in Human Experimentation," *Texas Reports on Biology and Medicine*, Vol. 32, No. 1, Spring, 1974.

Chapter II

[1] A more complete account of this case is given in Naomi Remen *et al*, *The Masculine Principle, The Feminine Principle and Humanistic Medicine*, San Francisco, 1975, pp. 67-81.

[2] See also the working definition of humanistic care, in Dr. Barbour's paper, pp. 50-52.

Chapter IV

[1] See Barbara Bates, "Doctor and Nurse: Changing Roles and Relations," *New England Journal of Medicine,* Vol. 283, No. 3, July 16, 1970, pp. 129-134; Sister Charles Marie Frank, *Foundations of Nursing*, Philadelphia and London, 1959; and Susan Bowan-Ferres, "Loeb Center and Its Philosophy of Nursing," *American Journal of Nursing,* Vol. 75, No. 3, May, 1975, pp. 810-185.

[2] Beatrice Kalisch, "Of Half Gods and Mortals: Aesculapian Authority," *Nursing Outlook,* Vol. 23, No. 1, January, 1975.

[3] Jerome P. Liysaught, "From Abstract into Action," *Progress Report From The National Commission On Nursing And Nursing Education,* Vol. 20, No. 3, March, 1972, pp. 173-179.

[4] Roberto Assagioli, *Psychosynthesis: A Manual of Principles and Techniques,* New York, 1965, and *The Act of Will,* New York, 1971.

[5]For an introductory annotated bibliography of readings in humanistic psychology for health educators and other health professionals see, R. Blau, *et al, Cases and Methods in Humanistic Medical Care,* San Francisco, 1975, pp. 96-103. The two works by Brown on confluent education cited in Chapter I above provide a general introduction to the principles and methods of that approach.

[6] See the discussion of an expanded understanding of the person in Sara Miller's paper following, pp. **68 - 69.**

Chapter V

[1] Both diagrams are adapted from Roberto Assagioli, *Psychosynthesis,* New York, 1965, p. 17, and *The Act of Will,* New York, 1973, pp. 13 & 14. The diagrams summarize the results of Assagioli's synthesizing large areas of modern psychology and are more fully explained in his two books.

[2] For a full exposition of this concept and its roots in traditional and psychological thinking and research, see Stuart Miller, "Dialogue with the Higher Self," *Synthesis,* Vol. 1, No. 2, pp. 120-139 and Roberto Assagioli, *Psychosynthesis,* pp. 17 et passim and *The Act of Will,* pp. 223-224 et passim.

[3] See the case of Harold, described by Dr. Remen, in Chapter II.

[4] Robert Hoke, "Healths and Healthing: Beyond Disease and Dysfunctional Environments," paper presented at the Annual Meeting of the American Association for the Advancement of Science, Washington, D.C., 29 December, 1972, p. 11.

Chapter VI

[1] See Allen Barbour's and Sara Miller's discussion above and Naomi Remen, Raymond Hively and Anita Astrom Blau, *The Masculine Principle, The Feminine Principle and Humanistic Medicine,* San Francisco, 1975.

AUTHORS

ALLEN B. BARBOUR, M.D.

Dr. Barbour is Professor of Clinical Medicine at the Stanford University School of Medicine, where he has been Chief of the Division of Ambulatory Medicine since 1963. For the decade before that, he was in the private practice of internal medicine in San Rafael, California. He graduated from the University of California Medical School in San Francisco in 1943. For most of the thirty years he has practiced internal medicine, he has been a consultant and teacher, as well as a primary practitioner. He has sought to achieve a comprehensive approach to patient care, with a particular interest in psychosomatic medicine.

DALE GARELL, M.D.

Dr. Garell is a pediatrician who is Chairman of the Department of Pediatrics at Mount Zion Hospital in San Francisco, California. He trained at the University of Colorado Medical School and the University of California at San Francisco. He became a Diplomate of the American Board of Pediatrics in 1965, and took fellowships in adolescent medicine at Children's Hospital, Boston, Massachusetts, and in social research at Bedford College,

University of London, England. From 1963 until 1973, he was Director, Division of Adolescent Medicine, Children's Hospital of Los Angeles, and Associate Professor of Pediatrics at the University of Southern California. He is past-President of the Society of Adolescent Medicine, and is Chairman of the Committee on Youth of the American Academy of Pediatrics. He serves on the Editorial Board of the American Medical Association *Journal of Diseases of Children*. He has made numerous published contributions to the field of pediatrics and adolescent medicine.

SARA UNOBSKEY MILLER, M.A.

After completing her graduate training in special education in 1963, Mrs. Miller served as a special education teacher in schools and reading centers in several New York communities, and developed and directed pilot programs in innovative education. She was Assistant to the Director, Community and Special Education Department, Coney Island Hospital; and then Director of Special Education, Demonstration Center, Yeshiva University Graduate School, New York. In her recent work she has served as Director of the three-year Ford Foundation Confluent Education Research Reading Program (University of California, Santa Barbara) and Director of the two-year Ford Foundation Confluent Education Program for School Administrators (University of California, Santa Barbara). She has been consultant to numerous agencies and organizations and is currently Director of the Institute for the Study of Humanistic Medicine.

STUART MILLER, Ph.D.

Dr. Miller studied comparative literature at Yale University and served as Assistant Professor of English and Comparative Literature at Berkeley and Rutgers University, and as Associate Professor of Literature at State College at Old Westbury, New York. In addition to teaching and research, he has worked to find humanistic alternatives to contemporary higher education in a variety of administrative posts at Berkeley, Rutgers and Old Westbury. He served as Editor of the Viking Press Book Series in Humanistic Psychology. His published books include *Measure, Number and Weight: A Study of the College Grading Problem* (University of Michigan); *The Picaresque Novel* (Case Western Reserve University Press); and *Hot Springs* (Viking Press). He is currently Director of the Institute for the Study of Humanistic Medicine, and Editor of the journal *Synthesis.*

MARGUERITE ABELL NAKLES, R.N.

Mrs. Nakles is Vice President, Patient Care Services, at Marshal Hale Memorial Hospital, San Francisco. She graduated from Mercy College of Nursing in San Diego in 1960, and later received her Bachelor of Science in Nursing from the University of San Francisco. She was Assistant Director of Nursing Services at St. Mary's Hospital and Medical Center in San Francisco for six years, and has held her present position for three years.

NAOMI REMEN, M.D.

Dr. Remen is a pediatrician who is presently Director of In-patient Services and Coordinator of Medical Education for the Department of Pediatrics, Mount Zion Hospital, San Francisco. She graduated from Cornell Medical School in 1962 and completed her House Staff training in pediatrics at the New York Hospital/Cornell Medical Center, in 1965. Between 1965 and 1967, she was a Fellow in Pediatric Metabolic Disease at the Stanford Medical Center. From 1967 until 1974, she was affiliated with Stanford as Assistant Professor and Clinical Assistant Professor of Pediatrics, and as the Associate Director of the Pediatric Clinics. Dr. Remen is a Fellow of the American Academy of Pediatrics and is a Diplomate of the American Board of Pediatrics. She is a principal author of *The Masculine Principle, The Feminine Principle, and Humanistic Medicine.*

THE INSTITUTE

The Institute for the Study of Humanistic Medicine conducts research and development activities in the area of humanistic medicine. Results are disseminated through training courses, publications, consultations, educational materials, and a network of cooperating institutions in the United States and other countries. The Institute is non-profit and tax exempt. Further information can be obtained by writing the Institute for the Study of Humanistic Medicine, 3847 Twenty-First Street, San Francisco, California 94114. Telephone (415) 285-2854.

book design

JOHN NAKLES